ALZHEIMER'S DISEASE

Understanding the Disease and Managing the Challenges

JACK A. KLAPPER, MD
AMY KLAPPER GREAVES, EMT, MBA

Printed in the United States of America
First Printing, 2019

ISBN: 978-1-54397-044-9

The Mile High Research Center
1155 E. 18th Ave.
Denver, CO. 80218
www.milehighresearchcenter.com

TABLE OF CONTENTS

This book is dedicated to all of the patients and caregivers that have participated in research studies with us over the years. Thank you for being brave, proactive and dedicated to finding better treatments for this disease. Thank you for sharing your stories with us. We have learned so much from you.

ABOUT THE AUTHORS

Jack A. Klapper, MD is a Neurologist who began doing clinical research in the early 90s. After years of studying all Neurologic conditions, he became focused on Alzheimer's Disease due to the urgency he felt in finding a better treatment than what is currently available. He is the Director and Principal Investigator at the Mile High Research Center in Denver, CO; a private research center dedicated to finding new treatments for Alzheimer's Disease.

Amy Klapper Greaves, EMT, MBA is the manager and clinical research coordinator at the Mile High Research Center. She and Dr. Klapper have worked together on research studies for over 20 years. Her focus is on helping caregivers and participants live better lives with Alzheimer's Disease. Her time spent listening to the challenges of Alzheimer's Disease and researching solutions has led to the discovery of many solutions to daily living problems that help with every stage of the disease. Taking a holistic approach to the health of Alzheimer's patients as well as their caregivers, is the most important part of her work.

ALZHEIMER'S DISEASE

Understanding the Disease and Managing the Challenges

This book provides an opportunity to learn about Alzheimer's Disease. Our goal is to share scientific information and offer practical ways to address an Alzheimer's diagnosis and ways to work through the challenges Alzheimer's presents each patient and caregiver. We have been dedicated to research and assisting in the treatment of patients and families dealing with Alzheimer's Disease for many years. We are hopeful that our experience from a scientific perspective and from a practical perspective, will help you as you live with this disease and its difficult life changes.

Dementia is defined as deteriorating mental function. Alzheimer's Disease (AD) is the most common cause of dementia. It was first identified by Alois Alzheimer, a German Neuroanatomist and Psychiatrist who performed an autopsy in 1906 on a 50 year old female patient he had followed for 5 years. The patient had memory loss, sleep disturbance, and progressive confusion. Examination of the brain tissue under the microscope showed distinctive structures that Alzheimer called plaques and neuro-fibrillary tangles. In the 1980s the plaques were found to be composed of a protein called Beta Amyloid and the tangles to contain a protein called Tau.

For many years, the diagnosis of AD could only be confirmed by autopsy showing these plaques and tangles. Currently, the diagnosis can be confirmed by finding beta amyloid and/or tau on radiological images of the brain using a special dye or tracer which attaches to these proteins. It's also possible to find the same proteins in the spinal fluid by a lumbar puncture procedure. This procedure involves a needle placed between the lumbar vertebrae and withdrawing a small amount of spinal fluid is collected. This diagnostic method is much less expensive than a diagnostic PET scan.

A PET scan of this kind currently costs between $6000 and $10000 depending on the area of the country and the imaging facility used. Insurance will likely deny payment for this expense because there is currently no effective treatment for AD. This should change as soon as an effective treatment becomes available. A spinal fluid exam will cost around $2000. Again, this test will most likely not be covered by insurance. Spinal taps can be a little uncomfortable for a short period of time during needle insertion and a transient headache may follow the test.

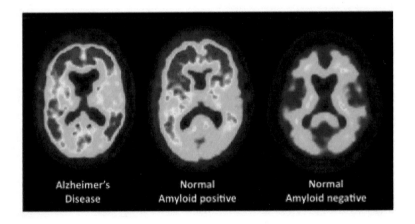

Photo credit: Jagust and Yang

The image above shows beta amyloid deposits on a PET scan using the specialized tracer. The red areas of the brain show the highest amount of beta amyloid. The middle image shows beta amyloid deposits in a patient who is not yet symptomatic.

An MRI scan is frequently used when patients are having memory problems to differentiate causes of dementia. MRI scans in patients with AD may show atrophy, or shrinkage of brain tissue, but this is not diagnostic of AD. The plaques and tangles associated with AD do not show up on a traditional MRI, and there are no other diagnostic features seen on the MRI. When atrophy is shown on an MRI scan, it can be helpful as a part of the diagnostic evaluation, but in and of itself, is not diagnostic of AD. This is why a PET scan or lumbar puncture in addition to the MRI is needed. Atrophy is measured by comparison to the average normal appearance of the brain in a similarly aged, non-demented patient. MRIs can be helpful to follow the progression of AD showing increasing atrophy over time.

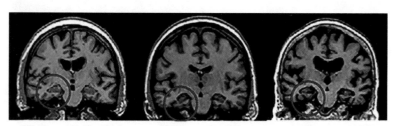

75 year old Control   75 year old MCI   75 year old AD

Photo credit: Dominique Duncan
(MCI: Mild Cognitive Impairment)

Atrophy in AD begins in the temporal lobe of the brain, as shown in the middle image. As the disease progresses, the atrophy becomes more generalized as shown in the last image. There is a noticeable decrease in brain tissue in the 3rd image and increased size of extracellular space or black areas.

An MRI scan, can and should be used to exclude other causes of dementia. Most insurance will cover the cost of an MRI during a diagnostic evaluation of dementia by a physician. Other causes of dementia include vascular dementia, Lewy body disease, frontal temporal dementia, normal pressure hydrocephalus, Creutzfeld-Jacob Disease and Chronic Traumatic Encephalitis.

Differentiating Types
of Dementia

Vascular Dementia

Vascular dementia is characterized by impaired judgement, difficulty planning, slow gait and poor balance, as well as declining memory. The MRI of a patient with vascular dementia would show evidence of multiple infarcts, strokes or bleeding in the brain caused by trauma. Patients with vascular dementia often experience transient ischemic attacks (TIA) as well as completed strokes. By definition, patients fully recover from a single TIA within 24 hours. Patients who have multiple TIAs may experience lasting memory problems and may not be aware of the causal connection between TIAs and memory loss.

Lewy Body Disease

Dementia with Lewy bodies often begins with sleep disturbance and visual hallucinations. Lewy body disease or DLB can be associated with Parkinson's Disease (PD). DLB usually occurs later in the disease progression in PD and can be differentiated from AD because of the Parkinson's symptoms. Dementia in PD is caused by changes in different areas of the brain than those affected by AD. Behavioral changes in PD dementia, such as hallucinations and delusions are similar to AD, but in PD dementia these can also be side effects of medication used to treat PD. If there are symptoms that are present in addition to memory decline, such as tremor, difficulty walking, and slowed movement and rigidity, a Neurologist should be consulted to differentiate PD from AD. An MRI scan will show changes in diagnostic areas of the brain that are the hallmark of PD.

Frontal Temporal Dementia

Patients with frontal temporal dementia (FTD) , previously known as Pick's Disease, show early personality and behavioral changes such as apathy, lack of empathy, trouble controlling behavior and overeating. Memory is usually spared early in the course of the disease. MRIs of FTD patients show a distinctive pattern of atrophy in the frontal and temporal regions of the brain. The onset of FTD may be seen between the ages of 40- 50, which is earlier than the average age of a person diagnosed with AD. A person with FTD may have a more rapid decline than an AD patient.

Normal Pressure Hydrocephalus

Normal pressure hydrocephalus (NPH) can occur after an infection or hemorrhage in the brain and is characterized by difficulty walking and controlling urination as well as memory problems. This disease has a distinctive diagnostic pattern on a MRI or CAT scan. It's possible to treat NPH with a procedure to shunt the spinal fluid from the brain to the vascular system, which may relieve the pressure. This procedure has complications and is not always successful.

Creutzfeldt-Jacob

Creutzfeldt-Jacob Disease(CJD) is a rare and rapidly progressive disease with behavioral changes characterized by problems with coordination, memory decline, muscle jerks and increased reactivity to external stimuli, such as loud noises. This disease is thought to be caused by an infectious protein contracted by use of contaminated surgical instruments or tissue from animals with CJD. The abnormal protein in CJD is called a prion. In CJD, this prion is a misfolded version of a normally occurring protein, which the body can not eliminate. Recent studies have suggested that misfolding of the Beta Amyloid protein occurs in AD.

Chronic Traumatic Encephalitis

Brain trauma can cause cognitive deficits, but these are not progressive and therefore, are distinguishable from AD. Significant trauma to the brain is however, easily distinguishable on an MRI. Athletes who suffer multiple concussions, or brain injuries, may develop a condition called chronic traumatic encephalopathy (CTE). CTE is characterized by memory problems, depression, suicidal ideation and personality changes. In the cases of CTE that have been autopsied, the pathology is quite different than that of an AD brain. In patients with CTE there are tau deposits located in the frontal/temporal region of the brain. Unlike AD, patients with CTE have very little beta amyloid deposits.

What We Know About How Alzheimer's Disease Starts and Progresses

---

The onset of recognizable symptoms of AD can occur in patients as young as 50 and the frequency of the disease increases with age. The earliest symptoms include difficulty with short term memory, word finding problems and difficulty completing complex and multi-sequenced tasks. Some physicians use the term Mild Cognitive Impairment (MCI) in the early stages of the disease to refer to patients who are able to maintain independent activity in all areas of their lives. These mildly affected patients are aware of declining memory and cognitive performance and are beginning to require assistance in daily tasks that have become too difficult or frustrating to perform independently. When patients get to this point, the diagnosis shifts from MCI to Mild AD.

The type of cognitive symptoms seen in any given patient depends on the parts of the brain that are involved in the pathologic changes (deposition of beta-amyloid and tau). The earliest changes are seen in the dominant (left side in a right-handed person) temporal lobe of the brain. This is the area of the brain that has to do with memory. As the disease progresses other symptoms are seen.

Scientists have determined the beta-amyloid spreads from the temporal lobe by moving from brain cell to brain cell much like an infectious particle. When the frontal lobes become involved, the patient's ability to plan and organize diminish. If the parietal lobe is involved, word finding, speaking and understanding conversations can be impaired. The spread to the parietal and occipital (posterior) areas of the brain can cause problems with visual-spatial orientation and result in difficulty maneuvering in ones environment. The medical term for this is apraxia.

An occasional patient maybe severely impaired in most areas of the brain, but may show accurate musical memory. This suggests that the non-dominant (right temporal lobe in a right-handed person) is relatively unimpaired. Early life memories (termed long term memory) are retained better than short term or recent memory.

Evaluating Cognitive Impairment

Cognitive impairment is most often evaluated on a scale called the Mini Mental Status Examination (MMSE). This is a 30 point memory test that targets short term memory, word finding difficulty, sequential task completion, simple mathematical calculations, ability to recreate geometrical patterns and orientation to time and place. A perfect score on the MMSE is 30 out of 30. A mildly impaired patient in the early stages of AD would typically score between 24 and 30 on this test. As the disease progresses, a moderately affected patient would score between 18 and 23, and severely impaired patients score below 17. Patients in this later stage of the disease usually require assistance with activities of daily living such as dressing, bathing, eating, toileting etc.

Performance on the MMSE and other cognitive tests can be adversely affected by several variables including test anxiety, lack of sleep, and medications for pain or anxiety like opioids, narcotics, tranquilizers or muscle relaxants. It's sometimes appropriate to repeat the test if it's suspected that these factors played a role in the outcome of the testing.

The MMSE is the standard of care for AD diagnostics and follow-up. More complex neuropsychological testing is time-consuming, expensive and emotionally draining for the patient. In our experience they do not change diagnosis or AD treatment and is not usually necessary.

It is not surprising that many diagnosed AD patients are depressed because of their loss of cognitive ability. In addition, AD may directly impact those areas of the brain that are involved in the disease of depression. Depression questionnaires and other diagnostic tools are helpful in evaluating whether or not depression is present and how it should be managed. Along with evaluation of depression, suicidal thoughts and plans need to be monitored on a regular basis by physicians and family. In current AD research studies, a suicidality questionnaire is administered at every visit. These questions include whether or not the patient has been considering suicide and if they have a plan in place. Changes in suicidal thoughts can happen suddenly and oftentimes without the awareness of close family members. For this reason, we recommend periodic evaluation of suicidal thoughts for all AD patients. These questions can be uncomfortable and caregivers can request physicians take the responsibility to ask these questions of the patient if they are being seen on a regular basis. If this relationship with a physician is not in place, it's important for the family to start the conversation and continue it to ensure the safety of the patient.

Being Diagnosed: A Blessing or A Curse?

In 2011, the National Institutes of Health and the Alzheimer's Association revised and clarified their diagnostic guidelines for AD. One of the additions was to add a phase of the disease called Mild Cognitive Impairment or MCI. Many people experiencing mild short-term memory loss receive this diagnostic. Doctors and patients may use the term MCI as opposed to mild AD because AD has a negative connotation. We feel this negative association is due to the tragedy of witnessing or learning about the decline of a loved one who had AD. However, our experience with clinical trials in AD suggests that there are medications on the horizon that show promise in extending or improving quality of life for those living with AD.

A patient may be relieved to receive a diagnosis of MCI rather than AD. In our experience, however, MCI is an early phase of AD and should be acknowledged accordingly.

The MCI diagnosis must include all of the following symptoms:

- concern about a change in cognition relative to previous functioning

- impairment of one or more cognitive functions, like memory and problem solving, that is greater than expected for the person's age and education. (Memory is the function most commonly impaired among people who progress from MCI to Alzheimer's dementia.)

- preserved ability to function independently in daily life, though some complex tasks may be more difficult than before

- no dementia

The only difference between an MCI diagnosis and an AD diagnosis is the 3rd criteria – preserved ability to function independently in daily life. That means that if handling one's finances was always challenging, but recent cognitive issues have made it so difficult that the task needs to be given to another family member or professional. This would change the diagnosis from MCI to mild AD. As discussed previously, there are other forms of dementia besides AD and differentiating them requires imaging scans at this point in time. A simple blood test that will be diagnostic of AD is being evaluated.

The problem with receiving a diagnosis of MCI is that there are no current treatments approved for this particular stage of the disease. Many people will benefit from using the standard of care prescription of a combination of Aricept and Namenda. However, with only a diagnosis of MCI in an individual's medical records, insurance companies have been quick to deny these treatments. In addition, many patients can spend years, in this phase of the disease. At some point, their caregiver might want to start working on getting a Power of Attorney in preparation for decisions they will need to make in the future. We've seen caregivers have a very hard time obtaining a Power of Attorney without their loved one having the full diagnosis of AD. Doctors can add a clarifying statement to their diagnosis, calling it Mild Cognitive Impairment due to AD.

This may seem like semantics, but it can be helpful as caregivers and family members approach important decisions that will need to be made. Sometimes the diagnosis of MCI can be the reason better care is not provided. If this is the case for you, you can ask your provider to make a clarification. It's also important to keep the provider updated on any tasks that the AD patient has turned over to the caregiver, as this should change their formal diagnosis.

Genetics in AD

Many patients with AD have another family member that was experienced similar symptoms, whether or not it was diagnosed as AD. This raises the question of a genetic link. In the 1990s the APOE gene was shown to be associated with AD. This gene has 3 sub-types; APOE2, APOE3, and APOE4. The APOE gene directs the cells to make proteins. These proteins help the body clear the Beta Amyloid deposits. The APOE4 sub-type is the least efficient of the sub-types in clearing beta amyloid. Genes are located on chromosomes and every person receives 1 form of the gene from each parent. It's possible to have one or two sub-types of the APOE4 gene. Having 1 type of APOE4 increases the risk of developing AD by a factor of 2-3 times the normal rate. Having 2 types of APOE4 gene increases the risk of developing AD 12 times the normal rate. It should be noted, that having 1 or even 2 copies of the gene does not necessarily indicate that AD is inevitable. Conversely, one can develop AD without any copies of the APOE4 gene. Clearly, there are other genetic factors that increase the likelihood of AD in addition to APOE4 that have yet to be discovered. It has been shown that people with 2 APOE4 genes have an earlier onset of the disease and are less responsive to currently available treatments. Testing for the APOE4 genotype is commercially available and can be ordered by your doctor. That test is done by a routine blood draw and can cost around $200. Depending on the insurance provider, this test may be covered.

Adult children of patients with AD often wonder if they should be tested for the APOE4 gene. Some people are reluctant to have this test because they feel a positive APOE4 result will cause unnecessary anxiety because there's no current treatment. We feel that it is important to know if you have an increased chance of getting AD so that you can plan accordingly. We would also encourage those genetically at risk to monitor new developments in the diagnosis and treatment of AD. Currently, there are studies underway for those who are APOE4 positive and have a family history of AD, but have not yet developed significant memory loss themselves. It is important to determine whether treatment of those with increased risk for developing AD will result in a lower incidence of the disease. Ideally, when effective treatments to clear beta amyloid become available, those who are positive for the APOE4 gene would take them preventatively. These studies are currently underway.

There is a large family in Columbia that has a genetic form of Alzheimer's Disease. This is different than the genetic link to APOE4, in that it is inherited as a dominant gene. This means that if they have just one copy of the gene, they have 100% chance of developing the disease at some point in life. This has provided scientists with a unique opportunity to study the early development of AD. Researchers can identify their genetics, and then study the course of the disease over time. It has been discovered that beta amyloid deposits occur in these at risk family members as early as 10-20 years before symptoms develop. Based on this finding, it is presumed that we will be able to diagnose patients at risk for AD long before they develop memory loss. We predict that it will become standard practice to determine APOE4 status and beta amyloid build up prior to the age when their family members began to have symptoms.

A similar form of AD has been found in the United States that is known as Autosomal Dominant Alzheimer's Disease (ADAD). ADAD is not very common. It can be distinguished by an earlier age of onset and multiple family members with the disease.

Regardless of one's genetic makeup, the rate of decline of AD is not linear. There may be long periods of plateau, and months of what seems like severe decline, only to return to a slower rate of decline, or a new plateau. When caregivers put expectations on what loved ones should be able to do because they did them the day or the week before, they set themselves up for confusion, frustration and even anger. Many find meditation helpful to release this tension. Meditation requires us to come back over and over again to the present moment, following each breath and releasing each thought. You might want to practice deep breathing, letting go, living in the now, and remember how powerful this moment is. It is the only place to be – everything else is unknown.

The Importance of Sleep

———

Over the years, the number of discussions we've had with patients and caregivers about sleep disturbances was hard to ignore. Now that research has focused almost entirely on the early diagnosed patient, we ask about sleep problems before our patients or their families bring them to our attention. Most have not put the two together. Almost all of our patients have a long history of poor sleep habits. There is a proven assosciation between sleep apnea and AD and many of our patients have this diagnosis. Some do experience an improvement in their memory and general functioning with treatment for sleep apnea. Many other patients do not have sleep apnea but nap frequently during the day and wake in the middle of the night, with difficulty getting back to sleep.

A normally functioning brain clears beta amyloid during deep sleep or slow wave sleep. This function might start to break down far earlier than the onset of signs and symptoms of AD . There is also evidence that as the disease progresses and the deposits of beta amyloid become more significant in multiple areas of the brain, the plaques of beta amyloid itself are interfering with the sleep-wake cycle. Many believe they can achieve better sleep with the help of over the counter sleep aids like Melatonin or Tylenol PM or prescription medications like Ambien. Unfortunately, these medications may interfere with the brain's ability to clear beta amyloid, although it is not known how this happens. More research is needed to determine if sleep disturbance causes beta amyloid deposits or is a result of them. However, evidence suggests that because sleep disturbances were present well before the AD symptoms began, it might very well be a big contributing factor to the formation of plaques. In one study, a single night of sleep deprivation led to a significant deposit of beta amyloid and one night where a significant amount of deep, slow wave sleep occurred, resulted in a clearing of the same amount of the protein.

Recently, two studies showed that a reduction in non-rapid eye movement (REM), slow wave sleep, and sleep deprivation, was associated with an accumulation of the tau protein in people with normal cognition or very mild cognitive impairment. Adding to this research, we know that tau deposits, which make up the tangles in the brain in AD patients, are correlated with cognitive decline, even more so than beta amyloid. It wasn't clear whether the tau deposits caused the sleep disturbances or the sleep disturbances led to the tau protein deposits.

A Few Tips to Promote Good Quality Sleep

We suggest starting a nighttime routine to prime the body for deep sleep. The first and probably most important step of this routine starts during the day. Walking for 15 minutes 3 times per week is enough exercise to slow cognitive decline and more vigorous activity shows no additional cognitive benefit. The National Institutes of Health (NIH) also suggests moderate exercise for 20-30 minutes during the day, improves circulation and blood flow to the brain, boosts brain cell production, turns on adrenaline and endorphins, and gives the body a natural rhythm of exertion that will result in a natural rhythm of rest.

Exercise can be something that couples do together. Going for a walk, or doing an exercise class together can be fun and a great way to stay connected. Any activity that is fun and gets the body moving is recommended, although being outside for a 15-30 minute walk can be the easiest thing to do and has the benefit of adding exposure to the sun, which has been proven to be helpful in promoting good quality sleep. There are also many ways to exercise at home with videos on the internet, but the more AD patients engage with their community, the better they do. Local recreation centers that offer group classes can be a great way to get connected to new people and form a routine that is fun and motivating. Any kind of activity that is enjoyable enough to become routine is the best. If they once played tennis but haven't picked up a racket in years, it might be time to return to the sport and find some friends that want to play. Choose something that you will look forward to doing. Physical activity is very important when dealing with the decline of AD and can be a great release for the stress and frustrations that come with this disease.

After a regular exercise routine, the nighttime routine should be easy and enjoyable. Keep dinner a very light meal so that the body is able to digest it easily. Avoid eating 2-3 hours before bed, even longer if possible. Shut down electronic devices at least 30 minutes before bed and again, even longer if possible. In the precious time before going to sleep, choose a few steps that will help your mind and body wind down physically and emotionally from your day. Take a bath, light a candle, read a good book, or find a great meditation that you connect to and do that for 5, 10, 15 or 20 minutes. There are many good meditation apps available as well as YouTube videos. Find a voice that is soothing and peaceful. This voice will become your guide so this is quite important.

For some, meditation may be the key component to holistically wiring the brain for optimal function. Turing off the constant flow of excessive worry and over-thinking that locks us in anxiety, depression, even inaction, is a necessity for optimal sleep. Both patient and caregiver can benefit from this practice. Meditation takes us out of living in the past, which creates depression and out of the mind space of the future which creates anxiety, and it brings us into the here and now. This is so important for the caregiver. Think about all the times you go into memories of what used to be with your loved one. Those are the moments we can easily keep going back to and the emotions that result can be so painful. It's almost like a papercut that you can't stop touching even though it's just as painful every time you touch it. This pain needs to be felt and shifted in some way. If you can share memories with others, or write them down, sometimes this helps move through the pain. It's as though these memories need to be given a voice or a permanence to mark their importance.

Other times we can find memories that make us laugh through the tears. Humor is an important factor in the well-being of the patient. We see this time and time again in couples and families that find a way to shift the pain into laughter. The goal is not to hide the pain, but to move through it to a lighter way of seeing things. In our experience, those who can move toward humor, experience less rapid decline and an easier course of the progression of the disease. It's interesting that so many patients maintain their good senses of humor throughout the course of the disease, even when many of their other mental capacities and pieces of personality have been lost. Others develop a fantastic sense of humor their family members say wasn't there or wasn't as good before the disease symptoms started. Humor seems for many to be a natural protective device patients use to deal with this painful disease.

Many times AD patients struggle with waking in the middle of the night and not being able to go back to sleep. This can cause a lot of daytime sleepiness and napping which can in turn interfere with the next night's sleep and cause the cycle to continue. If this is a problem, a meditation and deep breathing practice can be really helpful and can shorten the time awake significantly. Applying a good quality, organic lavender essential oil to the temples and taking 2-3 drops in your palms, rubbing your hands together to activate the oil, and taking deep inhales of the scent can help as well. Diffusing lavender oil by the bed can be helpful and using a home-made linen spray with water and a few drops of the oil misted on the sheets is a good idea as well.

It's important to avoid electronic screens when waking in the middle of the night as they are proven to extend wake time for at least 30 min once the eyes adjust to them. Reading with a small book light can help if the patient is still able to enjoy reading. The less one does physically in the middle of the night, the better the chance of getting back to sleep quickly.

In addition to these suggestions, the NIH has proven the following suggestions to be helpful in helping AD patients sleep better:

- Limit the intake of stimulants such as caffeine or tea

- Naps longer than half an hour or after 1 pm should be avoided.

- Time in bed during the day should be reduced.

- The schedule for going to sleep and getting up must be regular and the bedroom should be reserved only for sleeping.

Every person taking care of an Alzheimer's patient will tell you that each day is different. If we don't come to understand and accept this, it can lead to frustration. We have to learn to take each day as it comes. The road of decline in Alzheimer's disease is slow and bumpy. The average AD patient lives for around 10 years after they are diagnosed. The range is variable because some people are diagnosed early in the course of the disease perhaps because they had family members who had AD and they recognized the changes fairly early. Others aren't diagnosed for years after their symptoms become apparent. Many people live quite successfully hiding their symptoms from people at work and even family members. It may be that these people have developed mechanisms to cope with their early AD symptoms such as leaving themselves notes and catching themselves before they make mistakes. We have noticed a trend in a certain sub-set of patients who have always lived functioning at an extremely high level in all areas of their lives. These patients tend to decline at a much slower rate than those who perhaps didn't push themselves to their cognitive limits throughout their lives. There may be some legitimacy to the idea of treating your brain as a muscle. Those who have continued to exercise their cognitive functions have developed and neuro-connections that will result in a slower progression of the disease. We suggest continuing to learn new things, reading, and socializing for optimal cognitive function.

Alcohol, Sugar and Inflammation

___

Many caregivers and patients are surprised to learn that even one alcoholic drink per night can affect their cognition. One drink in a person sensitive to alcohol can be detrimental to cognition. Alcohol is toxic to human cells. We know this effect can be permanent. We recommend patients that are really motivated to do everything they can to improve their memory, stop drinking alcohol. Some might find this too restrictive, but alcohol is converted to sugar in the brain and we know that an excess of sugar is associated with inflammation in the body and is counterproductive to optimal brain health. We have long known that inflammation is present in brains of those with AD. We don't know if inflammation is the root cause of the disease or the body's response to the excess deposits of beta amyloid and tau proteins. We do know, however, that neuro-inflammation leads to more and more damaged neurons which can lead to the onset or worsening of AD.

Excess alcohol can lead to changes in the intestinal wall allowing bacteria to move into the blood stream; a condition called leaky gut, which triggers inflammation. Patients with AD are already susceptible to inflammation. Deposits of beta amyloid peptides and tau proteins are highly insoluble and thus result in inflammation. The question remains, is inflammation a part of the disease process or the result of the insoluble proteins presence?

There is definitely a higher risk of AD in patients diagnosed with diabetes. The primary source of fuel for the brain is glucose. Diabetics do not process glucose efficiently and therefore brain cells are not getting the fuel that is needed for their proper function. Because of this link, researchers have tested insulin in AD patients. Unfortunately, it was not successful in treating memory loss.

We can say that nearly every AD patient we have treated over the years has a sweet tooth and it would be fair to say most have a sugar addiction. As their disease progresses, many lose the ability to self-regulate their sugar intake and over-indulge on it. Caregivers are then forced to keep processed sugar products out of the house. Processed sugar isn't good for anyone and there are links to a high-sugar diet and cognitive decline. A study of 5,189 people followed over 10 years found that those with high blood sugar showed a faster rate of cognitive decline than those with normal blood sugar levels. Participants in this study did not have blood sugar levels that were diagnostic of diabetes. Higher carbo-hydrate intake is correlated with an increased risk of AD. This is one reason why a Mediterranean diet that is lower in carbohydrates and processed sugar is recommended for patients with AD.

There is some evidence that people with rheumatoid arthritis have a lesser risk of AD. This research comes from Denmark where the country keeps health data on all its citizens. This has led to clinical trials of anti-inflammatory medications as treatment for AD, but unfortunately, they have been unsuccessful.

Different parts of the world have different prevalence of AD. For instance the Mediterranean area has a lower incidence which has been attributed to diet. The Indian subcontinent also has a lower incidence than the U. S. which some attribute to inclusion of curcumin, a component of the spice, turmeric, in the diet, known to have anti-inflammatory proper-ties. Some people have begun using only the active ingredient, curcumin to help treat inflammation and memory loss. However, to maximize the effect, one must ingest turmeric in its complete form rather than just the curcumin because curcumin by itself does not lead to the associated health benefits due to its poor bioavailability. Others have suggested that coconut oil might have improved some patients' cognition, but we are not aware of any controlled studies which confirm this. Of course, controlled dietary studies are very difficult and expensive to perform. Consuming turmeric and coconut oil as part of a healthy diet might very well be helpful. Excessive doses, however, could cause side-effects. We would recommend using turmeric as part of healthy diet rather than taking turmeric supplements, because we aren't absolutely sure of the correct effective and safe dose in many of these products.

Hearing Loss and Memory Loss – There is a Link

Much like the link between poor sleep and memory loss, most people aren't aware of the link between hearing loss and memory loss. The research is fairly new, but it is impossible to ignore. Relevant studies have shown that treatment of hearing loss in AD patients with hearing aids or cochlear implants results in significant improvement in cognition.

Hearing loss can be isolating and when patients can't hear well, they have to work a lot harder to understand what others are saying. This may cause fatigue and lead to patients "tuning out" what others are saying, which can then lead to less cognitive activity. Decreased cognitive stimulation can increase the rate of AD decline. In addition, AD itself my cause damage to the area of the brain responsible for auditory comprehension and hearing. The important thing is to correct hearing deficiencies as soon as they are noticed to prevent associated cognitive impairment and social withdrawal.

Driving

Another question that will inevitably arise is when is it time for the person with AD to stop driving? In this area, it doesn't make sense to wait until the signs of concern are obvious.

There are too many unfortunate stories to tell, but the one we use to help families understand how important tackling this issue is before it gets out of control, involves a fairly mildly affected patient. He was starting to get lost driving outside of his neighborhood, but his wife and adult children didn't want to take away his freedom to run errands around a 1 mile radius near his home on a regular basis. In their minds, this was safe. One morning, the man took a routine trip to the grocery store and on his way out of the parking lot he was involved in a 3 car accident. He was certain the accident wasn't his fault, but he was confused and disoriented at the scene. When the police came to take the report, they noted this individual's confusion. The insurance company for one of the people involved in the accident was notified of this and they were able to request his medical records. Because of his diagnosis of AD, he was blamed for the entire accident, lost his insurance, and had a great amount of guilt and shame.

It's understandable that this is not a conversation a caregiver wants to have with a patient. Driving is associated with freedom, and even control over one's life. It is especially difficult for adult children to have this conversation with a parent. The authority role is reversed, and it can be uncomfortable. When we talk to caregivers about the importance of being proactive and not waiting until the first accident to have this conversation, they usually cringe and groan. We always offer to take this off their plate and have the doctor discuss it with the patient.

Another option if your doctor doesn't offer this help, is to talk to your insurance company and explain the situation. They would be happy to discuss this with the patient and explain that their decision to stop the driving is based on the diagnosis, not the actual driving ability the patient has at the moment. It's important to remind patients that changes usually happen gradually, but on any given day, there could be a lapse of judgment which is common in mild to moderate AD. This could easily result in an accident and they could hurt someone or themselves.

We have occasionally had patients very curious to know if they are actually having driving issues and want unbiased proof of where they stand. It is always an option to go to the Department of Motor Vehicles and ask for a competency test. It's important to remind everyone that there are many drivers on the road who are texting, unfocused, or impaired with drugs or alcohol. If they hit your loved one and are at fault, blame might be placed on the individual with AD simply because of their diagnosis.

Once the shock of this reality sinks in and the anger or loss has been felt, we've seen many patients become very relieved at not having to drive. It's clear there was a certain amount of stress and fear that went along with driving, that they might not have fully been aware of at the time. Driving services like Lyft and Uber have become a new way of finding freedom. The cost of driving services is minimal in relation to paying for monthly insurance and car maintenance. In short, take action before an accident happens. The price of waiting could be high and is completely avoidable.

When Will I Know When It's Time for my Loved One to be in a Memory Care Facility?

———

We have been asked this question more times than we could count. The answer has evolved to be, "you will know." There will come a time when there is no question remaining. These moments are different for each couple or family but they usually fall into 3 categories: safety concerns, physical aggression, and bowel incontinence. The first scenario occurs when the patient can no longer be safe alone in the home for even a short period of time. We have had examples when stoves were left on, water left running and overflowing the sink, or the front door left open and the patient is gone, wandering the streets in confusion.

Many caregivers have overcome some of these obstacles with solutions that made it possible for them to continue to care for their loved ones at home. We have one resourceful caregiver who found a company that makes a device that automatically turns off the stove if it hasn't been touched for 30 minutes. This fix helped, but it was only one part of the problem. Despite the stove no longer being a concern, it became clear the patient was becoming more and more anxious every time he was left alone. This caregiver eventually hired a company called Visiting Angels, the perfect name for this type of company. They have lovely, helpful people who the patient has enjoyed getting to know. These individuals keep the patient company while his spouse is out. This has resolved the safety and anxiety issues and this caregiver continues to be able to care for her husband with the help of these visiting angels.

If you are resourceful, including financially resourceful, there are options for keeping loved ones at home for the duration of the disease, however there are other examples of problems that need to be considered.

Physical aggression is common, especially in male patients in the moderate to severe stage of AD. There are patients who have kept a lid on their aggressive tendencies their whole lives, only to lose this protective mechanism in the later stages of AD. These episodes can change from aggressive words, temper tantrums and fits of rage to actual physical aggression even though they might not have ever had this kind of extreme aggression before their diagnosis. We have occasionally seen patients who never previously showed aggressive behavior, suddenly have a violent episode that frightens the caregiver and family members. If, and when this happens, it is a sure sign that professional assistance is needed. This is a red line and unfortunately, there is no going back and it will likely happen again. Isolated episodes may occur if the patient is having a reaction to new medication, short on sleep, out of his comfort zone or very anxious.

There was one patient, a retired policeman, who had been traveling back and forth across the country visiting family who had recently had a baby. The patient was showing many signs of stress and anxiety because he was out of his normal routine and comfort zone while away. His family didn't realize how much it was affecting him. One night, he got up in the middle of the night, and went outside for a walk. He was in the alley behind his daughter's home when a neighbor, who didn't recognize him, called the police. The patient was so confused when the police began questioning him, he became aggressive and pushed one of them away from him. He was promptly thrown to the ground, handcuffed and taken away to spend the rest of the night in jail.

The story doesn't end there. When the couple returned home, the patient began to hallucinate that his old police force owed him money and he had to settle the debt, in person. He would demand every day that someone take him down to the station so he could get his money. He never became physically aggressive again, but his hallucinations and fixation on getting this imagined debt paid, lasted for 5 months after they returned home and got back to their routine. It was an incredibly difficult time for his entire family, but eventually he returned to his baseline and the hallucinations stopped.

The importance of good sleep and routine in the AD patient can not be underestimated. If there are very unusual circumstances that one can pinpoint which would explain physically aggressive behavior, like this case, it might be wise to wait and see if the behavior subsides once the conditions return to normal. However, this is fairly rare and the vast majority of times, physical aggression is a problem that should not be ignored.

Bowel incontinence can show up fairly early in the disease for some patients. It's a sign that decline is happening more rapidly. The incidents can happen in the middle of the night or when the patient is out walking the dog, but they are always as disturbing for the patient as they are for the caregiver. Couples that have been married for decades have struggled the most with this problem. We've discussed with caregivers whether or not they feel their spouse would have wanted them to take care of this issue if they were able to go back and discuss it with them before the disease took hold. We also discuss if the tables were turned and they were the ones with the incontinence, would they want their spouse to be in charge of this, or would they want a trained professional to take this over this job? These are difficult questions, but when the time comes, you will know the answer that's right for both of you. While you may constantly question whether you are doing all you can for your loved one with AD, guilt has no redeeming qualities for the caregiver and we need to constantly remind ourselves of this.

Participating in Research

Most major pharmaceutical research in AD is focused on attacking the protein that causes the hallmark plaques in the brain of AD patients – beta amyloid. Many recent studies with therapies designed to either break up these plaques or stop the process by which this protein builds up, have failed. Some researchers are beginning to believe that treatments designed to attack beta amyloid or tau protein which makes the tangles in the brain of AD patients, are never going to work. They believe the research is targeting the wrong theories, although there aren't many other good theories on alternative treatments.

We have been doing these studies for many years and we have seen many promising therapies that have showed verifiable improvement on patients' mild to moderate AD symptoms that their caregivers, families and friends have recognized. When the studies ended, the treatments stopped, these patients often declined and lost the previously noted improvements. However, the tests used in the study did not show what was being reported to be seen in everyday life. The answer may lie in the cognitive assessments chosen by AD study over the last 20 years. These tests were not designed to target the newly diagnosed AD patient with mild symptoms. They ask questions that relate to more moderate decline and ask caregivers about such topics as eating, bathing, and other self-care problems that aren't evident in a mildly affected AD patient's life. They are so outdated that they ask about the patient's ability to use a phone book. These particular tests are a primary outcome measure, meaning it is the sole data point responsible for assessing a treatment's success or failure.

The industry is beginning to recognize these issues and a few have started using a new test that simulates going to the grocery store and forgetting one's shopping list – a perfect short term memory loss situation. We are very hopeful that this new test will objectively show what we are seeing subjectively in our patients' lives.

Often there are reports in the news media about the latest Alzheimer's discovery that is touted as a breakthrough. Unfortunately, these are predominately based on studies in mice that are genetically programmed to mimic symptoms and pathology of AD. Rarely do these results translate to viable human studies due to safety concerns or lack of efficacy. Results in animals do not necessarily translate to humans.

The day your loved one receives a diagnosis can be overwhelming. As we've noted, the current treatment options are only mildly affective. They do not slow the progression of the disease. We know the outcome of the disease with the current available treatment. It's hard not to go to a place of hopelessness. Participating in a research study of a new treatment can be a positive, hopeful way to proceed. There are studies currently in progress, and most large cities have a variety of research sites running these trials. You can find a list of studies at www.clinicaltrials.gov and filter your search for Industry AD studies.

Local Alzheimer's Associations provide a list of current studies within a designated area. This program is called Trial Match. The website for the Alzheimer's Association is www.alz.org. Often these research opportunities offer a positive experience for participants.

Many people call our office asking about our research only to say, "I don't want to be a guinea pig, I just wanted to know what you're doing." The people that volunteer to participate in AD research studies are those that are committed to doing everything possible to find a different path forward than those they've watched decline from this disease. Being a guinea pig isn't accurate of course, because animal studies occur in the first phase of research or Phase I which is much different than participating in Phase II or III studies that are the ones which test treatments on actual patients with the disease. In Phase I, animals and healthy human volunteers without AD are tested to see if the medications are safe and to find the dose that causes the least amount of side effects. By the time patients with the disease are studied, the medication has moved into Phase II and III. Phase II is to determine efficacy and the lowest possible effective dose. Phase III is long term safety and efficacy.

All phases of research must be approved by the FDA and the status of the studies is closely monitored for the safety of the participants. Research studies in the United States are also protected by Institutional Review Boards (IRBs). These boards are made up of a committee of health providers and respected community advocates such as clergy members and attorneys. These boards review all study protocols and safety data to protect participants and add an extra layer of protection of participants' rights and safety. Some IRBs will oversee an entire protocol for the country, and others will oversee specific research sites or hospitals involved in the research. A research participant is free to contact the IRB overseeing their study to discuss any concerns they have about the research site where they are being treated or other issues they might have with the study.

Our patients see themselves as being proactive in looking for treatment of their condition. They also feel a certain altruistic calling to move the research forward so that their children and future generations have a more hopeful future. After all, there is no clinical treatment advancement that can be made without volunteer participants.

The other thing to remember about participating in a research study, is that the study team is under strict guidelines put forth by the FDA to adhere to what's called Good Clinical Practice or GCP. Basically, under GCP, the health and safety of the research participant always comes first. That means, if there is any cause for concern regarding an abnormal lab finding, EKG report, or adverse reaction to the study medication, the study team is obligated to do everything medically necessary to care for those problems, regardless of the study protocol. Research participants are free to withdraw from a study at any time, as it is a purely voluntary role and there are never any costs associated with participation. All members of clinical research teams train and are certified regularly on GCP. If the guidelines aren't followed, the FDA can audit a research facility at any time and take action to stop their research if they are in violation of those guidelines.

We frequently get questions about privacy. It is not widely known that when one participates in a research study, the level of patient confidentiality and their privacy is greater than when one goes to see a doctor outside of research. The records we keep on participants are only identifiable by the patient's initials and date of birth. The research sponsor cannot see any other identifying information or they will be violating their government required privacy regulations. As the research team, we are not permitted to release results of study-related cognitive testing to any other physicians, insurance companies or other entities because they are proprietary to the research sponsor. If necessary, certain test results like blood work, EKGs, MRI or PET results can be released with the participant's written permission, but again they will only be identified by initials and DOB on these and all study related documents. Some participants do not want their insurance company, employer or other entity to be aware of their participation in a research study and there is no requirement for anyone to report their participation.

All good clinical research studies are placebo-controlled, meaning a certain percentage of participants will receive an inactive dose while others receive the active treatment. The percentages vary from study to study, but most often the split is either 1/2 of participants on placebo and 1/2 on active treatment; 1/3 on placebo, 1/3 on a low dose of active treatment, and 1/3 on a high dose of active treatment.

These studies will also always be blinded to the study team and the participants. This means that the doctor, research team, the patient and the caregiver don't know into which treatment group they have been randomly assigned. The idea is to keep everyone neutral to the outcome of the study and for the staff to not persuade the participants of a treatment's efficacy which could result in a positive placebo response and potentially skew the study results. Successful research studies rely on a separation of the placebo group response from the treatment group response. This means the placebo group follows a normal course of decline in memory during the course of the study, while the treatment group either maintains their baseline scores or improves. After all subjects around the world participating in the study have completed the placebo-controlled portion, most companies will "un-blind" the study and release the information about which treatment group each participant had been assigned to during the study. This can take years as these studies usually require a 2 year placebo-controlled phase and continue to enroll participants over a 2-3 years period until they reach their projected number of participants. Un-blinding usually happens a long time after most participants have completed this phase and have since moved on to an extension phase where there is no placebo and all participants receive an active dose of study medication.

Some participants don't understand why they can't be un-blinded once their participation in the placebo-controlled portion of the study is complete. The reason for this is that the study team cannot be un-blinded or we risk creating a biased atmosphere for all the participants who are still involved in the placebo-controlled phase. The company supplying the study medication also does not want anyone in the community discussing their positive or negative results from the study medication while the placebo phase is ongoing because of the potential to influence current or future participants or news outlets before the research is completed and analyzed.

Good candidates for research studies are generally healthy. That means that all current medical conditions are well controlled and medication doses are stable. The vast majority of AD studies exclude people who have had a recent heart attack (within the last 2-5 years depending on the study), cancer (within the last 2-5 years depending on the study), and all stroke and past brain injury. Stroke and brain trauma can result in cognitive impairment which is different from AD. Studies try to keep the cause of memory decline as similar as possible in all of their participants.

Other exclusions tend to be severe hearing or sight impairment that would interfere with the cognitive testing. Patients with bi-polar disease, major depression, schizophrenia that would interfere with these tests are also excluded. Epilepsy, Parkinson's disease, uncontrolled diabetes, heart disease and high blood pressure are excluded as well. Substance abuse, including alcohol is always excluded and often use of narcotic pain medication may be limited or excluded as well as use of marijuana because of the effects on cognition. Every study has its own exclusions, but these are the standard ones that seem to be on every protocol.

The Importance of the Caregiver in AD

In addition to being generally healthy, participants in these studies need to have a reliable caregiver that either lives with them or sees them 3-5 days per week and is familiar with intimate details of their daily routine. This is because they will be asked questions about changes in their eating, sleeping, bathing and general behavior that help research staff assess how the participant is doing. The caregiver's role in a research study is just as important as the participant's. They give us a glimpse into the patient's day to day life that the participant might not be able to assess him/herself.

At our research center, we have a dedicated enrollment specialist, who discusses enrollment criteria with potential research participants and assists them in getting their medical records to the doctor for review. The enrollment specialist goes through all the study specific inclusion and exclusion criteria with the potential participant. When the question of whether or not they have a caregiver that sees them regularly and can accompany them to every study visit is asked, it's surprising how many people say, "No". Family, friends and a strong tie to one's community are extremely important in the longevity and happiness of AD patients. The families that have a long history of unresolved emotional pain and then are faced with the consuming task of caring for a family member that caused or participated in the pain, understandably have the hardest time.

There are financial burdens, time burdens, and emotion care burdens associated with being an AD caregiver and these all can become a source of bitterness when faced with these old, unhealed wounds.

If there ever was a time for healing, a new role of being a caregiver for a family member with AD is the perfect opportunity for coming together. We've seen a lot of unkind words, manipulations, even cruelty between adult children who were previously hurt by their parent who now has AD and it's painful to watch. We have seen couples married for decades who were living to retire, travel and enjoy their later years, only to become bitter and angry because the diagnosis of AD has thrown a massive wrench in their plans. Newly married couples have it hard as well. We once had a woman call us in a panic to urgently get into a study because her fiancé had just been diagnosed and caring for him as newlyweds wasn't what she had envisioned.

When the caregiver is given a chance to voice all of the ways memory problems are affecting their friend/spouse/parent, it's always quite emotional. We have a tissue box ready in every room we conduct caregiver conversations. Often the caregiver is isolated or doesn't have the opportunity to freely discuss how difficult these situations are and they are grateful for the chance to be heard and to know they are not alone. We always recommend caregivers join a support group so they can meet others that are going through the same thing. Local Alzheimer's Associations are a great resource for these support groups; they also offer a host of helpful coping strategies for caregivers. Some don't want to go to hear people complain or to see a glimpse of what's to come if their loved one is not as far along in the progression of the disease as others in the group. Some chapters of the Alzheimer's Association have specific support groups for the newly diagnosed and the more advanced stage of the disease. There is often a good amount of problem solving that occurs at these meetings and people share their tips and tricks for some of the more confusing ways AD can affect people.

Solving the most frustrating problems that result from memory loss can seem impossible and the result of this thinking is endless frustration which can turn into resentment and later, regret. Sometimes, there are simple solutions that caregivers can't possible come up with themselves because they have a hard time accepting that the way their loved one is thinking has changed.

If a couple has always had a method for keeping their schedule, say on a large calendar in the office, this can suddenly become confusing for the patient and can result in arguments between the patient and the caregiver. The difficulty lies in the patient getting confused by a month's worth of engagements and appointments. The caregiver often thinks the patient is being lazy, annoying, not themselves. But as we discussed previously, apraxia can cause problems visually navigating the calendar and at a certain point this skill becomes impossible. Not being able to find the basic day's schedule easily causes anxiety for the patient, and the result is the repeated question of what are we doing today? This question, repeated 5-6 times an hour, can become unbearable for the caregiver who is just wondering over and over again why the patient doesn't check the calendar the way they always had. The patient needs to be able to see one day at a time, and probably to think one day at a time, one task at a time. We see over and over again that as patient's progress in AD, they begin to lose the ability to complete multiple tasks in the correct sequence. They complete the first step and leave the rest assuming it was done. Again, this can be very frustrating when we don't stop to remember that their brain is working in a new way and it's the disease taking over, not laziness.

A proven solution to the schedule problem is to get a small, inexpensive white board and write no more than 2 events for the patient to remember that day. Examples could be a doctor's visit at 9am, and lunch with kids at 12:30. That's enough. The white board should be placed in a frequently visited area like the breakfast table. Then, when the question of what we are doing today comes up, the caregiver can direct the patient to the white board to answer their question. This empowers the patient to find the answer to the question that is causing them anxiety and gives them an easy way to do it. If you make it a routine, it will get easier and easier. The AD patient thrives on routine and changes to it will result in anxiety.

Another very common complaint is neediness. Many spouses notice that their loved one's anxiety results in their wanting to be attached at the hip to their husband or wife. This can be especially hard when you love someone, but need your personal space. Some caregivers feel as though their loved one with AD has reverted to a toddler-like sense of neediness. They complain they can't even take a trip to the bathroom alone or without explaining that they will be right back. In these cases, it's so very important to get help.

Adult children, neighbors, visiting friends can become lifelines so that the caregiver can get some time to themselves. Many times, starting a weekly afternoon session at an adult care center that provides activities the AD patient enjoys can be a huge savior. Much like dropping a toddler off at day care for the first time, the AD patient might push back at the beginning, but they will adapt, become more comfortable, make friends and start to enjoy themselves.

We've also had couples decide to move into a senior living community so that friends are always nearby and activities are readily available for both the care-giver and the AD patient. Certain couples find this to be a mutually enjoyable decision. The Alzheimer's Association can help navigate the available senior living communities in your area.

Current Research Targets in AD

There is more research in AD being done today than ever before. These studies are being performed at large institutions like NIH, but also at regional hospitals, universities and private clinics. Most of these studies target beta amyloid and tau. Some medications being studied prevent the formation of these proteins and others are anti-bodies designed to block their activity in the brain. These medications come in pill form or are given by intra-venous injections at the clinic. There are other targeted proteins that are being studied as well. Almost all current studies target the newly diagnosed or early MCI/AD patients. There are some interesting studies being done on those at risk for the development of AD based on family history or APOE4 status and are currently asymptomatic. These studies attempt to prevent the development of the disease. There are studies currently being conducted targeting inflammation, excessive brain excitation and other theories. These studies can take years to complete.

Currently Available and FDA Approved Medications for AD

There are two classes of medication that are on the market and available for treatment at this time. One class is anti-cholinesterase medication which prevents the metabolism of cholinesterase which facilitates electro-chemical transmission in the brain.

The second class of medication currently available affects a different neuro-transmitter in the brain. There are multiple brand names for both of these classes of medications. They are available as pills, patches and extended release dosing. The two classes of medications can be used concurrently because they target different mechanisms. As with all medication, these drugs have possible side effects which can include primarily gastro-intestinal effects, hallu-cinations and dizziness.

Neither class of currently approved treatments for AD prevents the progression of the disease. They may improve quality of life to an extent and in our experience, some caregivers see an improvement in daily activities. They are certainly worth trying, but one should not expect major life-changing improve-ment with these treatments.

There are over 200 current AD trials currently in progress around the world. We are optimistic that more effective treatments will soon be available.

For more information about The Mile High Research Center please go to www.milehighresearchcenter.com. We are located at 1155 E. 18th Ave. Denver, CO. 80218. (303) 839-9900.